Acupuncture Treatment for Macular Degeneration:

Clinically Proven Methods to Recover & Preserve Retinal Health

Andy Rosenfarb, ND, L.A.c

Doctor of Naturopathy
Board Certified in Acupuncture &
Chinese Herbal Medicine

www.acuvisionacupuncture.com

MEDICAL DISCLAIMER: The following information is intended for general information purposes only. Individuals should always see their health care provider before administering any suggestions made in this book. Any application of the material set forth in the following pages is at the reader's discretion and is his or her sole responsibility.

What Patients Are Saying About Dr. Rosenfarb's Proprietary Treatment

No words can express my joy. Maintaining my eyesight means a normal life with complete independence. He and his staff are caring and professional, and I felt that the office was a home away from home. I believe that Andy Rosenfarb is as happy for me as I am. Thank you! —Fran

I came with hope to see Andy Rosenfarb, but expected nothing. After two weeks of treatment with acupuncture, herbs and micro current stimulation, my eyes have improved remarkably. —Edward

As I continued treatment, I noticed my vision gradually improving. It's great to know that my vision will not continue to deteriorate. —Jim

After a few weeks I noticed that I could see the TV better and I was bowling better. My scores are up and I continue to bowl with my friends. —Mildred

I noticed definite improvement and my vision improved in both eyes. My left eye was seeing 20/100 from 20/200. My right eye was seeing 20/400 and is now seeing 20/320. —Helen

Immediately after treatment I was able to drive 5 miles (through city streets) without my glasses. I found that I just don't use my glasses as much and end up leaving them around the house. —Mauro

My ophthalmologist said that a few years ago I was legally blind. After about 20 treatments I went back to my eye doctor and he said that he was very surprised to see that my eye sight had actually gotten better since he had seen me last. —Lillian

After 2 weeks of treatments, Andy was able to stabilize and return my father's eyesight back to what it was after treatment from the year before. The final result was that my father had no net loss of eyesight. Thanks to Andy, my father is healthier than he's ever been in his life.
-Son of elderly patient

After my first treatment I noticed a major improvement in my vision while driving home. The vision testing showed significant improvement in my vision as well. You are truly amazing. —Don

CONTENTS

5 GUARANTEES That You Can Bet The Farm On

- **You** won't find another acupuncturist more committed to your success than Dr. Rosenfarb. He'll give you 110%, 100% of the time.
- **You** will be treated like family, starting with booking the appointment, all the way to making sure you arrive home safely after treatment.
- **You** won't have the ball dropped on you. Our staff will take care of everything.
- **You** get your phone calls returned in 1-2 days and you will never have to "chase" us down.
- **You** get a team behind you that actually cares about you as a person, so we do everything possible to give you the best possible outcome.

FOREWORD

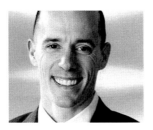

Greetings! I want to take this opportunity to thank you for taking the time to read the information I am about to present. If you are reading this book, you may have read about my work in Eye World Magazine or in the Johns Hopkins study. Either way, I'm glad you are here. I wanted to share a little bit more about myself and my passion for helping people with degenerative vision loss conditions.

Since 1997, I have helped literally thousands of patients with macular degeneration recover lost vision and help preserve what vision they have remaining. I specialize in working with patients dealing with various degenerative eye diseases. I really enjoy being there with my patients as they experience an increase in their vision.

I understand the commitment it takes when patients make the decision to travel to New Jersey to be treated by me. It's an honor and something I take very seriously. My team and I try to make the overall experience as enjoyable and comfortable as possible, all the way down to our weekly in-house workshops for our eye patients, their friends and family members.

Before I conclude, I do want to clear the air on a topic. **I understand that you may be skeptical.**

You may be asking yourself, "How can acupuncture actually recover your vision?" That's a good question and we will answer that question in this book.

Unfortunately, we have that there are many individuals who may try to discourage people with AMD from looking into treatment options like acupuncture. Many people have built up the courage to come and try acupuncture, are usually extremely pleased with the results they achieve. You will find some of their stories throughout this book.

Our goal here is to give you the best possible information we can about using our unique acupuncture methods to recover vision loss caused by Macular Degeneration. I have taken the top questions that I frequently get from patients and answered them in this guide.

With the exception of a few pages about us, this guide is all about you. Should you decide to book a treatment with us, we would be thrilled to have you join our family.

If you decide acupuncture isn't for you, that's fine too. We hope that you get value out of this book and all the free content we have on our website at www.acuvisionacupuncture.com

If I can do anything for you, please don't hesitate to contact me at my office.

In Health,

Dr. Andy Rosenfarb, ND, L.A.c.

What are the Main Causes of Macular Degeneration According to Chinese Medicine?

In Traditional Chinese medicine, the main patterns we usually see with age-related macular degeneration (AMD) are the result of internal blockages of Qi-energy and blood. Drusen is an ocular waste product that blocks the flow of energy and blood to the macula. Drusen (calcium and cholesterol) builds up in the eye are the first stages of macular degeneration and over time can impair blood flow to the macula causing slow starvation and suffocation, and eventually loss of function.

Your ophthalmologist will do a routine evaluation of your eyes and he/she will tell you if you have macular degeneration developing. "Qi" (Chee) is the universal "life-force" energy common in all living things. It's the animating, functional energy of the body. Qi-Energy can become blocked and/or depleted and degeneration may set in. Over time functional vision loss will progress and it will be more difficult to read fine print and eventually challenging to recognize faces.

When doing a Chinese Medical evaluation on patients with AMD, it is common to find an underlying liver and kidney weakness. This does not mean that you are in renal failure and/or have liver damage. It means that the adrenal glands liver detox pathways, kidney fluid and metabolism aren't functioning optimally. These metabolic processes can be the underlying cases for developing AMD.

Can Macular Degeneration be Improved?

Yes it can.

Being diagnosed with AMD can be a jarring experience to say the least. A person who has just been diagnosed with macular degeneration will tell you that their experience went something like this. "You're sitting in your chair and your doctor does this eye exam and tells you, "It seems as though you've got macular degeneration." Most people's response is, "What's that?" Your eye doctor may reply, "Well, it's an incurable eye disease and you're eventually going to lose your vision." What?

The next obvious question that most people ask is, "What can I do about it?" The conventional response from your doctor will most likely be, "Nothing". "You can take some AREDS vitamins and fish oil supplements, but there's really no conventional treatment at this time." -- meaning there is currently no drugs and/or surgery for AMD.

From a Chinese Medical and Naturopathic perspective, there's definitely a lot that we can do to recover lost vision, slow and/or arrest the degenerative process. The long term objective is vision preservation.

How Does Acupuncture Actually Work to Improve My Vision?

Recent research has shown that acupuncture increases blood flow to the eyes and stimulates different neurological areas of the brain. Through Ocular Doppler measures blood flow to the eye and research has shown that acupuncture can significantly increase blood flow to the eyes. Functional MRI testing shows that acupuncture can activate and suppress certain areas of the brain that are involved in visual perception. We can measure some of the effects of acupuncture, but at this point in time, we don't have a complete understanding of how the entire mechanism works. We definitely need more conclusive research.

At this point, all we know is that we see positive, measureable results with most cases. The results speak for themselves, and we are thrilled by the amount of people who have benefitted from this treatment.

What are the Chances to Recover Lost Vision?

About 85 to 90 percent of my patients have some improvement in their vision within the first round of 10 treatments. Generally for macular degeneration patients, there's some degree of distortion.

When patients first come in we test their vision. They'll read a certain line on the eye chart which is called their Baseline. Usually they will see an increase of 2 to 5 lines (or more) after 10 treatments. Those that are in really bad shape with advanced AMD can sometimes increase as much as 6, 7 or even 8 lines. Results depend on how far the condition has progressed and how much permanent nerve damage has been done to the macula. Dormant (sleeping) cells will wake up and vision improves. The vision that does not improve is due to either dead cells or scar tissue. The more dormant cells, the more vision will improve. It's impossible to know which cells are dead vs. which cells are dormant, until we start treatment which is why it's difficult to forecast precise gains for each patient. Some have more dead cells and others have more dormant cells.

How Do You Measure the Effectiveness of the Acupuncture Treatments?

This is a very important question. The key word here is MEASURE. Although I love hearing patients say, "Yeah, well, I think I see better," we need measurable results. We use conventional functional testing methods in our clinic like Amsler Grid, Visual Acuity and Visual Field Testing for our AMD patients.

In cases of macular degeneration, the central vision starts to go and people present with mild distortion to a total loss of vision in their central visual fields. Loss of central vision means that there's going to be difficulty with sharpness (HD vision), reading, as well as driving and face recognition. We'll look at these tests in order to determine the degree of functional vision loss. We also look at the results of the Amsler grid test, which is another functional test.

After the initial series of treatment, I typically send patients back to their ophthalmologists and their retinal specialists to get OCT and Fundus exams to monitor any physiological and structural improvements in the macula. We also want to see how the drusen is progressing (better, worse or the same). In summary, we use a combination of our in-house functional testing along with conventional ophthalmic testing as Third-Party-Confirmation that we have improvement and/or long term stabilization.

How Many Sessions Does Someone Need to See Results?

Most patients see measurable improvement within the first 10 treatments. Generally my patients come in for intensive daily treatments and we do 2 treatments per day for 5 or 10 days. Again, most patients will see some improvement within the initial 10 treatments, some severe cases may need the second week to see benefits.

How Long Will Treatment Last?

Benefits can last from a few months to a few years. Each case is different and factors like co-existing health issues, medications, diet, stress, lifestyle factors and compliance will play a role in how soon a patient needs to return for follow-up. Pretty much all patients will require some degree of follow-up treatment to maintain healthy blood flow to the macula. AMD is a neurodegenerative condition that is incurable. The best we can do is recover some lost vision and manage the condition to the best of our ability. Most cases I have worked with stabilize long-term as long as patients keep up with treatments, take recommended supplements and follow diet and lifestyle modifications.

Early stage AMD can benefit by receiving treatment every 1-2 years. When we're dealing with the more advanced stages of macular degeneration, patients may need to come in more often – two, three or even up to four times per year. On average, most of our patients come for maintenance twice a year.

Will Acupuncture Heal Macular Degeneration, for People in Their 90s?

80 to 90 percent of our patients respond well to treatment … at any age. You would think age would be a factor, but it seems not to be much of a factor in terms of overall response. I have found that factors like having other health issues, poor diet, sedentary lifestyle and high stress to be relatively more of an issue with rate of response. I have a patient who is in her nineties, and she's been coming for many years. She is doing great and maintains her vision and is enjoying life.

As long as a person still has light perception and if they can get to our office, there's potentially a lot that can be done in terms of improving and preserving vision. If there is no light perception, it's unlikely that treatment will be beneficial.

How does the Treatment of an Early-Stage Patient Differ From the Treatment of a Later-Stage Patient?

Generally, early-stage patients will have a much better prognosis because there usually hasn't been any nerve damage. The strategy of Preservation is a lot easier than cellular Resurrection and Resuscitation. The treatment is the same but because there is relatively more damage and the disease has progressed, it may take a bit more time to see improvements.

During early stage AMD, there's no nerve death and no visual abnormalities. As AMD progresses, there may be mild distortion. These patients will usually do very well because we see them at such an early stage. It's easier to prevent a fire than it is to put one out.

Later-stage patients will do great as well. It's just that there is a higher probability that there may be some degree of permanent damage from dead retinal cells and scarring. Again, each case is different and we just have to wait and see how each case responds.

Is There a Stage of the Disease Too Advanced for Acupuncture?

After treating patients for fifteen years, I don't believe any AMD is so advanced that treatment will not help. It's worth a try. Acupuncture can never make vision worse, it just not work in the worst case scenario.

Again, there are no significant side effects and no risks involved. It may take some courage and planning, but acupuncture is unbelievably safe. Acupuncturists pay about $700 annually for malpractice insurance. Some of my MD friends pay tens of thousands each year in malpractice insurance. Why the difference? Risk and side effects!

How Long Does the Recovery Process Usually Take?

First signs of improvement can be usually seen within the initial 10 treatments. Some more advanced cases may need a second course (10 more treatments). The dormant retinal cells recharge and we see an improvement almost immediately, usually within a couple of days. The regeneration of sick and/or damaged retinal cells can take between 8 to 15 months on average.

Nerve cells do regenerate but at a very slow rate. We have scar tissues/dead cells which, to the best of our knowledge, cannot be recovered and that damage is permanent. It's important to note that we don't know what is dead and what is dormant just by looking at the retinal cells in the back of the eye. We need to do acupuncture I order to wake up and stimulate the dormant retinal cells. Usually after about a year or so, whatever gains someone has made at that time is pretty much what you're going to have. Then we work on preserving vision long-term.

Would More Treatments Help Improve the Results Even Further?

People need varying degrees of treatment frequency and intensity. For macular degeneration and most neuro-ophthalmic conditions, maintenance is required in order to preserve vision. Think of it more as a marathon versus a sprint. We want short-term gains with long term preservation.

Each case is different and I create individual treatment plans based on your particular situation. More is not necessarily better. We don't want to over-treat, but we want to provide enough to facilitate a positive response and long term benefits.

I'll treat some patients two, sometimes even three times a day initially, just to see if we get a positive response. We want to get a clear indicator so as to see if the patient is a responder or non-responder.

I don't want to drag people along who may not respond to acupuncture; it's unfair and unethical to do so. If there is a positive response, we can continue; if not we go no further and the patient isn't charged.

More isn't necessarily better. For example, when we treat people for two weeks at a time, a lot of people are asking if they can stay for three, four or even five weeks. This is not necessarily going to help improve their situation. Why? In many cases, most of the significant healing occurs when the patient goes home. Remember, the initial improvement is seen when the dormant cells awaken. The sick cells take time to regenerate. The body needs that time to recover and regenerate healthy new macular cells.

We need a little time to rest because that's when our body recovers. We usually have patients come back sometimes six weeks or sometimes three months later for another round of treatment. That seems to produce the best results.

Are the Components of the Treatment Basically the Same for All Macular Degeneration Patients?

Every patient is unique. I do believe that protocols give SOME results, but they may only work to a certain extent and are limited. Acupuncture is not a "cook book" system of medicine. Knowledge and experience is critical especially when seeking out an acupuncturist to help you with your AMD.

The best results cannot be obtained without really addressing the underlying causes and the individual issues that are going on with each person. So we treat both the AMD and the underlying cause which is unique to each individual.

In all cases, we want to increase the blood flow to the macula and control the drusen deposits in order to maximize visual function. What's going on internally with each case differs from person to person. People have different stress factors, different health conditions and are on different medications, diets and supplements. We need to look at everyone individually and treat them as individuals in order to get the best possible results.

How Important is it to Find a Conventional Eye Doctor Who Acknowledges Acupuncture as an Effective Tool?

Whether or not your physician "approves" (or "disapproves") of acupuncture will not affect the outcome of our treatment. I do believe that it's really important to have a doctor that is ALWAYS supportive of the choices you make in order to try to better your situation – especially when there is no conventional treatment to offer. They should be your advocate and never give you a hard time. Of course, MD's are going to make appropriate recommendations based on what's available to them. This is all about YOU and your decision to take action in order to preserve your vision.

I recommend to all my patients that they find (and hire) an eye doctor (or any doctor for that matter) that has their best interests in mind. We all need a doctor who is really going to listen to you and put your best interest as top priority. If you want to engage in acupuncture and holistic integrative approaches, you may want to find a doctor who's really going to support that for you. It works better in my experience in terms of overall communication as far as getting additional testing done. It's a lot more of an open communicative, cohesive and positive experience for everyone.

Why Does My Doctor Seem to Dismiss My Questions About Other Treatment Options?

Retinal specialists, ophthalmologists and optometrists that I work with are great guys and gals, but frankly, they don't have much of anything to offer right now for patients with AMD. They will say, "Go take the AREDS and fish oil supplements which may help slow down the process".

Remember, most MD's operate in a relative "herd" mentality, which is reasonable in this day and age. This means that the Top Expert in a given field makes the calls regarding what all retinal specialists should be recommending to their patients. In short, they all follow an "industry standard" that most adhere to. Experimental and non-conventional treatments usually fall outside of that box. Physicians will probably know little to nothing about these alternative treatment options, therefore they are unable to give feedback and "dismiss" these treatment options.

I often hear my patients say, "I'm seeing the Top Eye person at this major university". I know that even the "top docs" are still doing the same as everyone else and following the same Industry Standard. Basically, no one does anything better or different than anyone else. They all test your vision and currently have no treatment to offer.

Most physicians today are in a difficult position and not free to recommend anything outside of what's customary within their field of specialization. Some eye docs may even consider making recommendations (like acupuncture) a risk. Is this because there are inherent risks involved with acupuncture? No, again it has more to do with the current legal system. A doctor can actually be sued for recommending something that is not conventional so to them, that's the real risk. Not worth it for them to lose their license, which is completely understandable. Our legal system is totally bananas, but that's another discussion. Just know that many of these docs have their hands tied in many situations.

Unfortunately, there are also those with big egos. To that I say, find another doctor who puts YOU before their own self-image.

Also, in their defense, they don't know much (if anything) about acupuncture and alternative medicine.

Right now the Conventional Industry Standard for the treatment of macular degeneration is the AREDS. Some also suggest fish oil and lutein and Zeaxanthin as well, but if you start asking about acupuncture, you may be hard-pressed to find a retinal specialist or eye doctor that is actually educated and can give you appropriate feedback. It's not unlike asking a plumber about marine biology.

Do what feels right for you and if it's something you want to pursue, do your own research and investigate all options that are available to you. Educate yourself and find an acupuncturist who has knowledge and experience treating AMD. There is a world beyond drugs and surgery.

Do You Educate Ophthalmologists and Optometrists on This?

Early on, I was kind of scared and intimidated that conventional eye docs were going to reject what I was doing. Some years later I had a real change of heart, having seen firsthand the consistent results that some were getting, and I chose to reach out to the medical community. I've visited with about 50 eye doctors in our area over the last few years, here in central-northern New Jersey and New York City and had the opportunity to connect with some amazing doctors.

I contacted them and said, "I'd like to meet with you and talk to you about what I do. I have some patients in your area and I want to make some referral and I'd like to learn more about you so I know who I am referring to." I just wanted to sit down with them and see if they had any cases that they could use my help with. Surprisingly, most were extremely open and receptive to my work.

Most of the eye docs were surprisingly interested in what I do and seemed relatively supportive of my work. I commonly heard feedback like, "We think this is really positive what you are offering for this patient's population, especially since we have nothing medical to offer at this point in time."

Of course, there will always be naysayers and some doctors who will say acupuncture is a "snake-oil treatment" or a scam. Often we hear things like, "You know it's not researched or proven to be effective." These folks are just hard-core cynics for whatever reason.

Going back, it's really incredible to me that just over the past five years or so, how many more conventional doctors have become receptive to this kind of work we are doing, including the researchers at Johns Hopkins University, NOVA Southeast and Retina India.

Can Conventional Treatment and Acupuncture Work Together for a Patient?

Absolutely. For example, a lot of our patients with wet macular degeneration are getting regular Lucentis™ or Avastin™ injection for retinal bleeding. Some patients are on blood pressure medications and cholesterol medications as well.

Integrative strategies do seem to provide the best possible outcomes for patients because we are really getting the best of both worlds. You are getting the knowledge and experience of a holistic, naturopathic and Chinese medicinal perspective, along with the cutting edge diagnostic treatment from conventional doctors can provide, Integrative Medicine provides optimal care.

Does Western Medication Lessen the Chance of Successful Acupuncture?

In my experience, it depends on the case and the type of medication.

I have had a lot of patients who have had Lucentis, Eyelea and Avastin injections for retinal bleeding. I think long-term there could be some damaging side effects because these are highly toxic forms of chemotherapy. Also, the body seems to build up a resistance to these meds. That needs to be considered and addressed by both the patient and his/her eye care specialist.

Drugs like heavy steroids and immune suppressants can nullify the effects of acupuncture.

Is Timing of Treatment Critical?

Absolutely! The earlier you catch it the better. The longer you wait the more probability of more severe or permanent vascular and nerve damage to the macula and the retina. The sooner you get treatment the better your chances for improvement and long term preservation.

There is no substitute for preventive medicine. Our goal is to try to recover as much vision as possible during the first year and then help you keep what you have for the long haul.

Do You Recommend any Adjunctive Therapies?

Yes. We often recommend adjunctive therapies such as micro current stimulation, eye exercises, acupressure, IV Vitamin drips and essential oils. There are also dietary recommendations, herbs and nutritional supplements. A lot of these strategies are outlined in my first book and they're on the website too. There are a lot of things you can do at home to be proactive.

Being proactive early on is a much better strategy than waiting until things get bad – when things get bad and your vision loss advances. I can't over-emphasize this point.

Can Hereditary Conditions Be Reversed?

I'm assuming that question is probably geared towards a condition called Stargardt's or Juvenile macular degeneration which is in the family of retinitis pigmentosa. This is considered genetic retinal disease. In my opinion, these conditions are usually rooted in auto-immune conditions and exacerbated by epigenetic factors. "Epigenetic" lifestyle, habits, environmental toxins and other stress factors. This seems to be the most probable underlying issues that influence gene switching and expression of this disease process. We have seen patients as young as four years old with Stargardt's Macular Dystrophy (it's real tough to treat some of these kids).

For these young kids, we usually use acupressure, micro current and low-level laser acupuncture treatment (LLLT) – no needles. These non-invasive treatments do not penetrate the skin and there's no pain what so ever. We get very good results with Stargardt and juvenile RP and Usher Syndrome, which are considered to be Genetic Retinal Diseases. LLLT seems to charge the Mitochondria in the cells and improve cellular ATP-energy output. It has also shown to improve ocular blood flow.

These conditions are a totally different issue than adult onset of age-related macular degeneration (AMD), which has more of a systemic cardiovascular disease as an underlying causative factor. The genetic conditions appear to be more of an auto-immune/auto-neurological disease that starts up relatively early on in life. We have had very good success in managing and preserving vision with these kinds of cases.

How Can Putting Needles in Someone's Hands, Feet and Forehead Help the Eyes?

We mostly stimulate certain acupuncture points in the hands, feet, back of the legs, etc. in order to improve the blood flow to the retina and macula. It kind of works like a light-switch. There is a switch on the wall that can turn on and off the light. You don't need to unscrew the lightbulb every time you want to turn on/off the light. The circuits and wiring in that wall connect the switch to the light. The same principles apply to the human body. We can turn switches (called acupuncture points) on and off that will affect different parts of the body. In this case we use points in the hands and feet which switch on the function of the eyes, increase blood flow and stimulate nerve activity.

Acupuncture also sends nerve impulses up to the brain to fire off the optic nerve, retina and specifically the nerve cells in the macula and waken dormant cells. Again, Acupuncture will dilate the blood vessels around the eyes and increase blood flow to bring food and oxygen to the retinal cells.

That's the short version of how it works. We are getting a neurovascular and physiological response from the acupuncture treatment from the needle therapy.

Is There a Limit to the Effect Acupuncture Can Have on Already Damaged Cells?

Yes, we can only wake up dormant cells, regenerate damaged or sick cells. There is nothing we can do for dead retinal cells. Once they die, they are lost forever.

After a period of 1-2 years of treatment, patients usually hit a plateau. They have been going for acupuncture treatment, taking herbs, getting acupuncture, making lifestyle changes and there comes a point when maximum recovery is obtained. Patients often wonder if acupuncture is no longer working, and if they should continue or try anything else. At this point we've completed the Second Recovery Phase of treatment and move into Phase 3 – Vision Preservation and Maintenance.

The other possibility is there may need to be a switch in the treatment strategy. Maybe using different acupuncture points, electro-acupuncture, or a different treatment strategy such as auricular acupuncture or laser acupuncture may help recover more vision. That may take your gains to another level to break out of the plateau stage.

In summary, there are two possible scenarios that are happening: 1) you are either going to plateau or reach maximum benefit or 2) it's time to switch strategies (or acupuncturists) and see if we can get further improvement or no improvement is made.

Should the Black Spots in the Center of the Eye Decrease?

A lot of people have floaters, which are little floating black spots in the vision. Acupuncture can certainly help with floaters. You don't have to have macular degeneration to have these either. If you do have floaters, that doesn't mean you're going to get macular degeneration. It's a very common occurrence and is generally nothing serious.

The floaters are debris made up of protein waste floating in the vitreous. The immune system should take care of this in a process called phagocytosis (white blood cells that are eating up the waste). The immune system improves with treatment and these cells eat up the floaters (waste), kind of like PAC-MAN gobbling up the ghosts.

When the phagocyte doesn't do this job, it can mean that the immune system could be suppressed and/or there's poor ocular blood flow. So these (AMD and floaters) are really two separate issues, but with acupuncture, the macula should improve, and the floaters should improve as well-both by improving overall ocular blood flow.

Is There a Relationship Between the Results and the Type of Macular Degeneration?

There are two types of AMD, wet and dry-type which are treated differently. Both respond very well to acupuncture, supplements, diet, exercise and micro current stimulation. Wet macular degeneration is a progressive state of dry AMD with the presence of neovascularization and retinal bleeding. Wet-type AMD consists of about 10% of all AMD cases and dry-type accounts for the other 90%.

In dry AMD, the eye accumulates drusen. "Drusen" is a lipid (and calcium) waste which clogs the macula and impairs blood flow. Over time, the macula will degenerate and lose its function from starvation and suffocation/oxygen deprivation.

The macula needs water, food, oxygen, and a clear detoxification pathway. In the body's wisdom, it will start to regrow new cells or "fuel lines" to feed the starving macula, which is an evolutionary adaptation for survival. These new blood vessels form in a process called "neovascularization". They are relatively weak blood vessels and very susceptible to breaking. When the blood vessels rupture, that's when you have the presence of "wet macular degeneration", which is bleeding in the retina. The bleeding could be short-term or it may become a chronic, long-term issue.

Dry macular generation is just the buildup of drusen over time, which impairs the blood flow and detoxification process of the macular cells. This results in the macula starving and suffocating over time. Eventually, the cells die and we lose vision if we do nothing to optimize circulation.

Imagine leaving garbage in your house and never taking the waste out. The accumulation of garbage and toxic fumes and rotting waste in the house would make the environment almost impossible to live in. That's really what is going on in your macula with AMD. The environment becomes too toxic for new stem cells to grow and thrive. When we have a toxic environment, we can't expect regenerative endogenous stem cells to be able to implant and mature into healthy retinal cells. We MUST improve the environment if we want to grow new cells and maintain health and function.

Is the Potential for Vision Loss the Same in Wet and Dry Macular Degeneration?

The potential for vision loss is much more serious with wet macular generation which is why the conventional eye specialists will do highly aggressive treatments such as Eyelea, Avastin™ and Lucentis™ injections. These drugs are chemotherapy meds that are highly toxic, but seem very effective in controlling bleeding for acute bleeds and retinal edema (fluids behind the eye).

It may take one or more injections of the anti-angiogensis meds to help the body absorb the blood and fluids so as to improve your vision. This is the standard conventional treatment for wet-type AMD, macular edema, and other kinds of retinal bleeding.

Does Micro-Acupuncture Work Better for Wet or Dry AMD?

Micro Acupuncture is a relatively new acupuncture micro-system. There are 48 newly discoverer points in the hands and feet. We have found that Micro Acupuncture is an extremely effective system for treating most degenerative eye conditions.

It works very well for both wet and dry AMD. We have seen pretty amazing results and about 85% see a measurable response within the first 10 treatments.

Are TENS or Electro-Acupuncture Bad for Wet AMD?

When administering electro acupuncture or micro current stimulation (MCS), you need to be careful with Wet AMD. There are a lot of people who do MCS for dry AMD, and get great benefits. If you are doing these types of treatments (a lot of local needling, or electro acupuncture, or micro current) you are going to increase the blood flow to the eye. We know that is going to happen and it may be too much for the weak blood vessels to handle. That being said, there is no substitute for an experienced acupuncturist who knows what they are doing in these kinds of situations.

If you increase the blood flow to the eye and you know there are weak blood vessels, you're really increasing the risk of retinal bleeding. This is why we use other distal points in the hands and feet as well as laser acupuncture.

Doing electro acupuncture or TENS on other parts of the body for pain, I haven't really found that to be much of an issue. I think you would be safe and not have anything to worry about with that.

If you are going to be doing anything around the head for something such as TMJ, I wouldn't do anything electrical with close proximity to the eyes unless you are experienced. The neck and shoulders are fine. If you are getting any kind of cosmetic treatment done, I think you should be ok.

What Can Someone Do Before Acupuncture Treatment to Improve Chances for Success?

Great question! A lot of patients ask me this before they come in to see me for treatment. They say, "What can I do to make sure that when I go get the acupuncture, I get the best results?" Here are a couple of things:

1) Stop smoking
2) Reduce Carbs and Sugars
3) Exercise daily
4) Eat lots of fresh fruits and vegetables
5) Increase your good fats like olive oil, coconut oil, avocado, nuts and seeds
6) Cut fried, greasy foods and pastries loaded with "bad fats"
7) Reduce alcohol, coffee and other stimulants
8) Take a good macular eye formula
9) Get adequate rest
10) Learn to better manage stress

Other things are to try to clean up your diet a little and make sure that you are well hydrated. People don't realize this but even things like drinking alcohol every day or drinking coffee is also very dehydrating to your body. The eyes are 95% water. When you are dehydrated either from alcohol or coffee, it may have a negative impact on your vision. Also a lot of excessive carbs, sugar, salt or junk food, and fried food can cause harm and accelerate cardio and neurovascular disease.

Make sure you're always well hydrated. Make sure you are taking electrolyte supplement if you are low in minerals and electrolyte salts (people with hypertension should use caution). Your overall diet should be pretty clean and "Heart-Healthy". No greasy fried foods and no trans fats. If you can, get aspartame out of your diet, which is present in many diet drinks, gums, mints, etc.

Get on a really good eye supplement. I'm really not a big fan of the Preservation and OcuGuard. There are a lot better formulas like MacuHealth Eye Formula. Mark Grossman has a great line of supplements as well at **www.naturaleyecre.com**.

There are a lot of great eye support formulas out there. Generally, get your body healthy. Reduce your stress. Get your sleep and clean up your diet a little bit. You want to make sure that you get the best possible results from your treatment.

By Treating Systematic Problems Prior to Treating Eye Diseases, Do Patients Get Better or Longer-Lasting Results?

Yes, absolutely! I wouldn't necessarily say we always have to treat it before we begin. For example, say somebody comes in with hypertension, has a gastric ulcer, or they have other digestive issues. We do treat both of these diseases at the same time because they are all symptoms that are intimately related to this person's systemic condition, which is causing AMD. Most of our patients with AMD are on cardiovascular medications (or will be in the near future) for hypertension and cardiovascular disease, or have a family history of cardiovascular disease. Some have other health issues going on but cardiovascular disease seems to be the number one underlying cause for AMD.

Through Chinese medicine and naturopathy, we can treat both AMD and the underlying causes at the same time. This seems to get long-lasting results and vision preservation.

Does Acupuncture Correct Organ Function in Order to Improve the Eyes?

Yes, acupuncture corrects the function of the organs as they relate to the specific eye conditions, in this case AMD. We call this "root and branch treatment". We treat the root (organ imbalance) and the branch (eye disease) in order to get the maximum benefit.

Our goal is to fine-tune this instrument called the human body, towards optimal health. We do that through acupuncture, exercise, diet, proper stress reduction, meditation, spiritual connection, friends, good relationships, and through listening to music. Anything we do will help the body to improve the overall health and function; will in turn have a positive impact on vision and it long-term preservation.

We have habits that can degenerate the organs, and the vision. I can do acupuncture long-term, but if somebody's going home and smoking cigarettes as well as drinking alcohol (on top of being stressed and not sleeping), at best we are going to keep it where it is at. We can't fight against these epigenetic lifestyle factors that will destroy health and function. My goal is to really help people see the whole picture here. To understand the impact of the lifestyle choices they make. We use acupuncture and all of our clinical resources to help people maximize and improve not just their eyes, but their overall health.

What Other Health Problems Should Someone Watch for in Order to Prevent Further Macular Degeneration Inflammation?

As I mentioned earlier, most patients with age-related macular degeneration have a family history and/or an existing cardiovascular disease.

People can be under the false impression that their cardiovascular disease is being controlled but when we see the accumulation of drusen in the macula this is (as seen in early onset AMD) in most cases it is linked to systemic cardiovascular and neurovascular disease. We know that because when you look at the back of the eye, you can see blood vessels and the buildup of drusen (cholesterol and calcium) that's going on in the retina. We can see that this is in the eyes and this is the only place we can actually observe what's going on with the vascular system.

It's simple, when we are treating people with macular degeneration, we are also preventing heart disease and heart attacks. That's one great side benefit to our treatment. Heart disease is, along with cancer and diabetes, among the leading causes of premature death.

By looking at the macula, we can identify cardiovascular disease early and control it. Thus, we help people preserve vision and over time, work on the heart as well. As a result, they may live longer, healthier lives as well as reduce medications they are on. The connection between AMD and cardiovascular disease is a VERY important observation that we've made.

What Else Can One Do Between Treatments to Help Retain Improvement?

Get the trans fats (donuts, cakes, cookies) out of your diet. Get the "Three Whites:" white sugar, white flour and salt out of your diet as well. I recommend that you eliminate gluten, and whole grains and sugar. Also eliminate greasy fried foods and all junk food.

Eat mostly organic vegetables, fish and lean meats. We also want to have good fats in our diets ... cholesterol is GOOD, not bad as we have been falsely led to believe. What's "bad" is low HDL's (good fats – and high LDL's (bad fats) along with inflammation. Good fats regenerate nerve tissue. So what do you think happens when we consume a low fat/no fat diet and take cholesterol lowering medication that destroy these fats? That's right! We no longer have the raw material (fats) that are used to generate nerve tissue.

So eat eggs, organic butter and milk (if you're not lactose intolerant), olive oil, coconut oil, avocado, nuts and seeds.

Exercising a little more and eat a little less. Reduce your body's BAD fat by exercising regularly and eating more protein, more good fats and more vegetables. Improve your lean body mass by cutting carbs, sugar and junk food.

It's also important for us to learn to better manage stress. We know that stress places a tremendous amount of extra work on the heart, brain and eyes ... and pretty much all the systems of the body. Reduce negative stress and focus on the positive things in your life. Spend more time with your family and friends. Work as you need to support yourself and your family but really try and balance your lifestyle with leisure and recreation. It is very important to audit your life regularly and make sure that you have a good work-to-play balance. Schedule regular rest and relaxation time for yourself and enjoy your hobbies as often as possible.

What Supplements Do You Recommend?

As far as supplements go, we are going back to the idea that each person is individual and must be treated as such. There are no supplements that are universal and work for every case of AMD – or any other heart condition. The supplements that I recommend help both eye and hart and preserve neurovascular and cardiovascular health and function.

I recommend supplements that help BOTH improve the macula, and supplements that address each individual person's underlying health issues. In order to figure out which supplements you are going to need for your own health issues, you should seek out an experienced practitioner. Either myself or somebody else who can help you understand your systemic issues and manage that, as it relates to your AMD.

As far as supplements that are going to be particularly beneficial for macular degeneration, whether it's early, mid-stage or advanced, research has shown that AREDS may help to slow down the process of progressive vision loss. This is basically Vitamin A, C and E, selenium and zinc are all good for eye health. Get on a good supplement, there are many out there. I'm not a big advocate of the Preservation or the OcuGuard as they are relatively inferior to other eye formulas on the market. They are manufactured by pharmaceutical companies which is why your conventional eye doctor will typically recommend those over other eye supplements.

Another great supplement is Resveratrol. Resveratrol comes from red grapes and red wine helps to digest unhealthy and excessive fats. There is a lot of research suggesting that Resveratrol may benefit the vascular system and overall hearth health. If it's good for cardiovascular disease, and heart health, it's going to be good for AMD. It seems as though Resveratrol may help break down cholesterol and drusen. Resveratrol is a good supplement for AMD.

There are some recent studies suggesting that a specific form of melatonin that can also help break down drusen as well. It also helps you sleep well. Sleep is critical for nerve regeneration and just overall health and we get the added benefit for reducing drusen accumulation

Lutein, Zeaxanthin and Meso-Zaxanthin are carotenoid antioxidants that are critical for retinal health preservation. I

Vitamin C is another supplement that is another supplement that is very important for AMD and heart health. Vitamin C is really important to support the blood vessels. There is a ton of research out there that shows how important Vitamin C is for cardiovascular health. The best form of Vitamin C is Liposomal/Lipospheric Vitamin C.

Which Foods Do You Suggest to Help the Eyes Heal From Wet AMD?

Colored vegetables and leafy green vegetables and fish are great. Keep your diet clean and organic if possible. Stay away from the junk food and fried foods. Vitamin K and a Chinese herb called "San Qi" (Notoginseng) can be beneficial for wet AMD.

In general, I recommend cutting out sugar and carbs. Add more good fats to your diet like olive oil, coconut oil, fish oil, avocado, sardines, eggs, nuts and seeds. We need fats to regenerate nerve tissue. Following a "low fat diet" is a very poor strategy for supporting eye health.

Is it Advised to Get Avastin Injections in the Eyes Every Three Months for Maintenance and Prevention?

I have mixed thoughts when it comes to Avastin™ and the other anti-angiogenic injections. I think the injections can be helpful in some acute cases of bleeding and edema. These are highly toxic drugs that are used for chemotherapy and can be very damaging to the sensitive structure of the eye. The pharmaceutical companies and medical community often recommend these injections be given every four to six weeks. They have increased recommended frequency from every three months to every month indefinitely. In my professional opinion, I think this is overkill and do not advocate this as a long term treatment.

I'm not going to tell people to take injections or not to, because I'm not a medical doctor and I can't do that legally. However, I do want people to understand what the injections are doing to the eye and the potential side effects. Do your homework and talk to your doctor about the risks involved.

We need to look at it and understand what these drugs do. Avastin™ is a chemotherapy drug originally used to treat colon and other forms of cancer. It is highly toxic to all cells of the body. It's also used for any form of retinal bleeding like diabetic retinopathy and other forms of retinal edema.

The goal of this chemotherapy treatment is to 1) mop up the blood and/or fluids and 2) destroy those new blood vessel growths in the eye, called neovascularization. These meds are so toxic that it's going to kill these new blood vessels, not unlike weed killer. These blood vessels that are growing I the retina in attempt to nourish and feed the starving macula. So the meds destroy the weak blood vessels and the macula still staves and the nerve cells die. The injections do NOTHING to support the health and function of the macula. In many cases AMD may even accelerate vision loss.

The injections may help stop the progression of the neovascularization (new blood vessel growth) but through what mechanism? Through increased cellular toxicity! You are actively poisoning the eyes and you're putting in these harsh chemicals in order to destroy the newly formed secondary blood vessels. If you are receiving injections every four weeks, what do you think the neurological and cellular consequences might be?

In my opinion, the long term side effects have not been researched enough and we don't know how damaging these meds can be. Is the drug accumulate to go into the brain and into the other parts of the body? We don't know how well the body can clear/detoxify these meds. How much medication is too much and how much each person can handle? What happens when patients develop a tolerance to these meds and bleeding continues?

What is the Comparative Success of Acupuncture to Eye Injections?

Again, our success rate is about 80 to 85 percent, meaning there are usually measurable results within the first 10 treatments. We don't really know about the drugs as far as their long term effectiveness (or harm). I don't necessarily trust the research in Avastin™, Eylea™ and Lucentis™ because the research is being done by the pharmaceutical companies themselves that are producing the drugs. There is an obvious bias and conflict of interest since the same companies that profit from the drugs are putting out the research. That goes for a lot of medications, not just these eye drugs. I don't know how accurately or honestly those research studies are being reported. These drugs are however the current medical standard of care for Wet-AMD and can be very useful in certain situations.

Again, keep in mind that with acupuncture we are working on both the bleeding/fluids and supporting health and function of the macula. This in turn will help preserve vision. Eye injections do nothing to improve the functional integrity of the macula. It's a band-aid treatment that is useful in emergency situations or when all other efforts have failed.

Is Your Technique Covered by Medicare and AARP?

Medicare currently does not cover acupuncture. I am pretty confident in the future it will be, within the next few years. I would say a lot of my patients with Medicare are submitting to their secondary insurance and getting reimbursed so a lot depends on your secondary insurance plan.

What is the Latest Conventional Research on Gene Therapy and Stem Cell for AMD?

Developments in Stem Cell and Gene therapy seems to be much slower than people are being led to believe, but some progress seems to be happening.

Pharmaceutical Researchers need funding and in order to get more funding they need to show that they are doing something seemingly productive. They present as if they are making progress and they get more money ... research is still a business that dies with income from funding and donations. Many people have a lot invested in these Gene and Stem Cell meds. Stem Cell and Gene Therapy research is Big Business.

Gene therapy works by "correcting the faulty gene" which will produce proteins that may result I genetic vision loss. Kind of like if you are building a house without roof materials. This therapy would be like "ordering" those missing materials so the job can be completed.

The issue here is dismissing understanding what is causing these mutations in the first place. Why not address the actual cause(s) rather than just addressing symptom? It's like trying to put out a fire while the house is still on fire. There are factors that altered the genetic coding and gene expression and most likely will continue to exist. Genes don't just change without a causative factor(s).

There are many concerns with stem cell, the primary being that stem cells migrate towards cancer cells which can result in tumor growth. Also, introducing too many stem cells to one area can cause unwanted tissue overgrowth. It's just so dangerous and uncontrollable at this point and time.

One other concept that may seem to be confused around Stem Cell (and Gene Therapy) is that these treatments will not recover lost vision and bring back dead cells. Researchers seem clear that (at best) they will slow the progress in order to preserve vision. In most cases, acupuncture does the same thing – without the associated risks. Acupuncture seems to facilitate regeneration and repair by stimulate Stem Cell Production.

There are two other major factors that Stem Cell researchers seem to be missing:

1) What is the underlying cause of the degeneration?
2) The environment (in the retina) has become so toxic and unhealthy that stem cells may not survive.

It's my opinion that the body has no shortage of stem cells in most cases. It's just that the environment (in the retina and macula) have become toxic and unhealthy over time and cannot support cell regeneration and regrowth. With disease breeding factors like inflammation, oxidation, acidity, low oxygen, and toxic accumulation of metabolic waste, it should be no surprise as to why the macula is degenerating and vision loss progresses.

So, what's the solution? Clean up the environment so healthy, new stem cells can implant and naturally generate. Get new freshly oxygenated blood that will deliver oxygen, food and other nutrients while removing the accumulated wastes. This will help to control acidity, inflammation and oxidation. Acupuncture, healthy diet, exercise, proper rest and supplements play a key role in maintaining an ocular and overall health. When the environment (our bodies and eyes) are healthy, damaged nerve cells will regenerate.

Stem Cell treatment is analogous to planting seed (stem cells) in the garden (retina). If the garden has no sunlight, no air, no nutrients I the soil and water being pumped in is toxic and dirty, will the garden grow? Of course it won't. There are certain conditions that need to be in place for the plants to germinate and grow. Our eyes need for optimal function and structural integrity.

One more point regarding research. I find it very curious (and concerning) that for the first time in history, people are being asked to fund their own participation in these kinds of studies. I have patients who have paid well over $20,000 out of pocket to be part of a research trial. Why?

I think that stem cell is amazing for certain conditions where there is acute nerve trauma. In that scenario, the environment is relatively unpolluted, so healing and regeneration is much more possible.

Once researchers better understand the importance of improving the environment, gene and stem cell therapy may work. I really do hope that they can figure that out and come up with a cure for AMD and other degenerative conditions. Until then, we need to be proactive and keep the remaining cells healthy and functioning. Once retinal nerve cells die, they are gone, there is no treatment that will bring back dead tissue. It's highly unlikely that science will resurrect dead tissue. Frankenstein is just a movie …

Certainly at this point acupuncture, proper diet, exercise and key supplementation, seems to be the best option going for AMD and Stargardt's. We need to control inflammation, oxidative stress and improve circulation and overall vascular health. There's simply no other treatment right now that's demonstrating the effectiveness that acupuncture and good nutrition can with zero side effects.

What to do Next:

Thank you for reading my book. I hope that you found it helpful in learning how acupuncture is helping people recover lost vision and preserve vision long term.

Now that you are armed with the information, you may be ready to take action. Here are your options. We hope you found the information presented in this book educational. If you reconsider in the future, we are available here to answer any questions you may have.

Option 1:

You have decided that acupuncture is not for you. No problem. You can now cross it off your list of treatment options.

Options 2:

You are still gathering information and have some questions that we didn't cover in the book. Be sure and check out the blog for some great free content, and also consider calling my office. This is a great way to get your questions answered.

Option 3:

You are interested in booking an appointment for treatment. Congratulations! I appreciate you trusting me with your vision. There is so much we can do to help you potentially recover some lost vision and help preserve what vision you have remaining.

For first time patients, we usually recommend 2 weeks of treatment. If that is not possible, we usually can determine a rate of response within one week. It will be done Monday through Friday.

All patients will have their vision tested before commencing treatment on the first day. Then we will test again after the initial series in order to confirm positive response rate. For those who want more in-depth eye testing than we offer, we encourage you to get vision testing before your visit.

To book a treatment, please call my office at your convenience and my assistants will work to get you on the calendar. We book months in advance, so don't put it off once you've decided to book an appointment. The sooner we get to work on preserving your vision, the better the probable outcome.

In good health,

Dr. Andy Rosenfarb, ND, L.A.c.

www.acuvisionacupuncture.com

908-928-0060

Made in the USA
Las Vegas, NV
08 August 2024

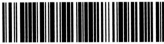

93538483R00040